I0447617

REFLUX AND VOMITING IN CHILDREN

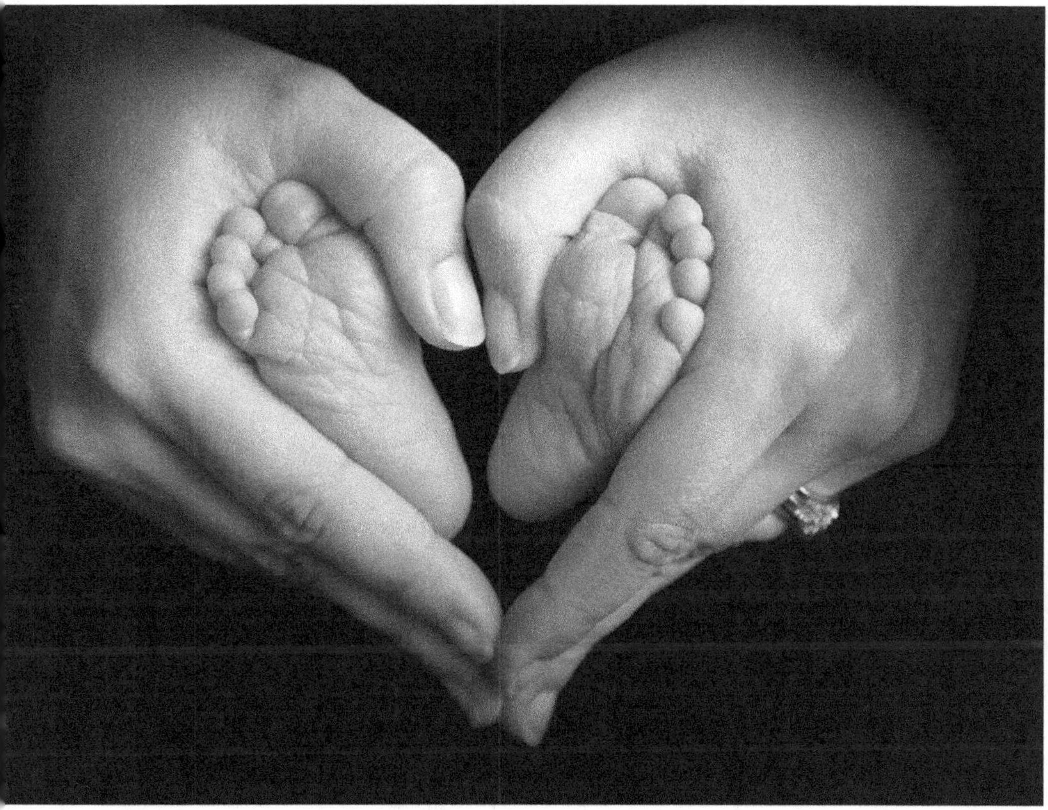

DR. NELSON J. SPINETTI

Copyright © 2013 Dr. Nelson J. Spinetti

All rights reserved.

ISBN-10: 1480005355

EAN-13: 9781480005358

Library of Congress Control Number: 2012919833

CreateSpace Independent Publishing Platform

North Charleston, South Carolina

TO MY WIFE, LIVANIA and children, Andres and Sabrina for the their love, understanding and support; to my parents and older brother for their love and support;

To my attendings Dr A. Kimbrough, Dr J. Udall, Dr E. Schmidt-Sommerfeld, Dr R. Brown and Dr D. Lagarde for the guidance, example as a leader in pediatric and pediatric gastroenterology and for inspiraring me to help others. To my office staff who are helping to deliver the care to my patients.

-NJS

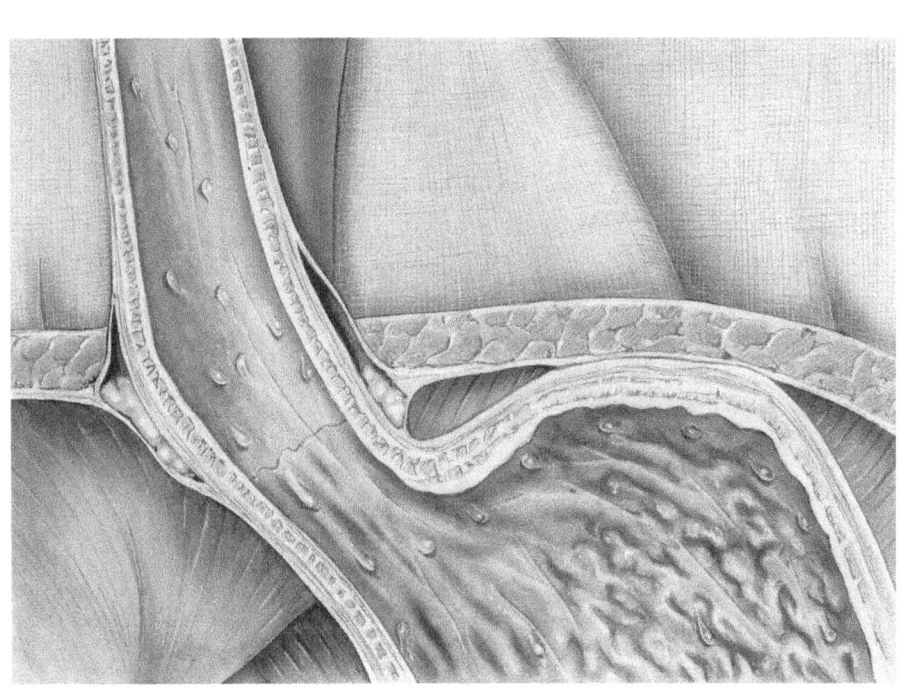

GASTRO ESOPHAGEAL REFLUX DISEASE

―――●●●―――

GLOSSARY

GASTRO ESOPHAGEAL REFLUX (GER): the return of gastric content into the esophagus several times over a twenty-four-hour period. These events could be considered normal in an individual if the episodes are short in duration, the natural mechanisms for reflux defense remain intact, and there is no subsequent inflammation or impaired calorie intake.

REGURGITATION: the passage of gastric content into the mouth.

SPITTING OUT: regurgitation which is expelled effortlessly through the mouth.

VOMITING: the forceful expulsion of gastric content through the mouth.

Vomiting is a complex symptom of GER disease as it is difficult to differentiate innocent GER from GER disease, because both conditions result in gastric contents being expelled through the mouth.

TRANSIENT RELAXATION OF THE LOWER ESOPHAGEAL SPHINCTER: a simple relaxation of the lower esophageal sphincter muscle or ring of muscles which is well recognized in healthy individuals and increases in frequency after eating due to increased gastric pressure.

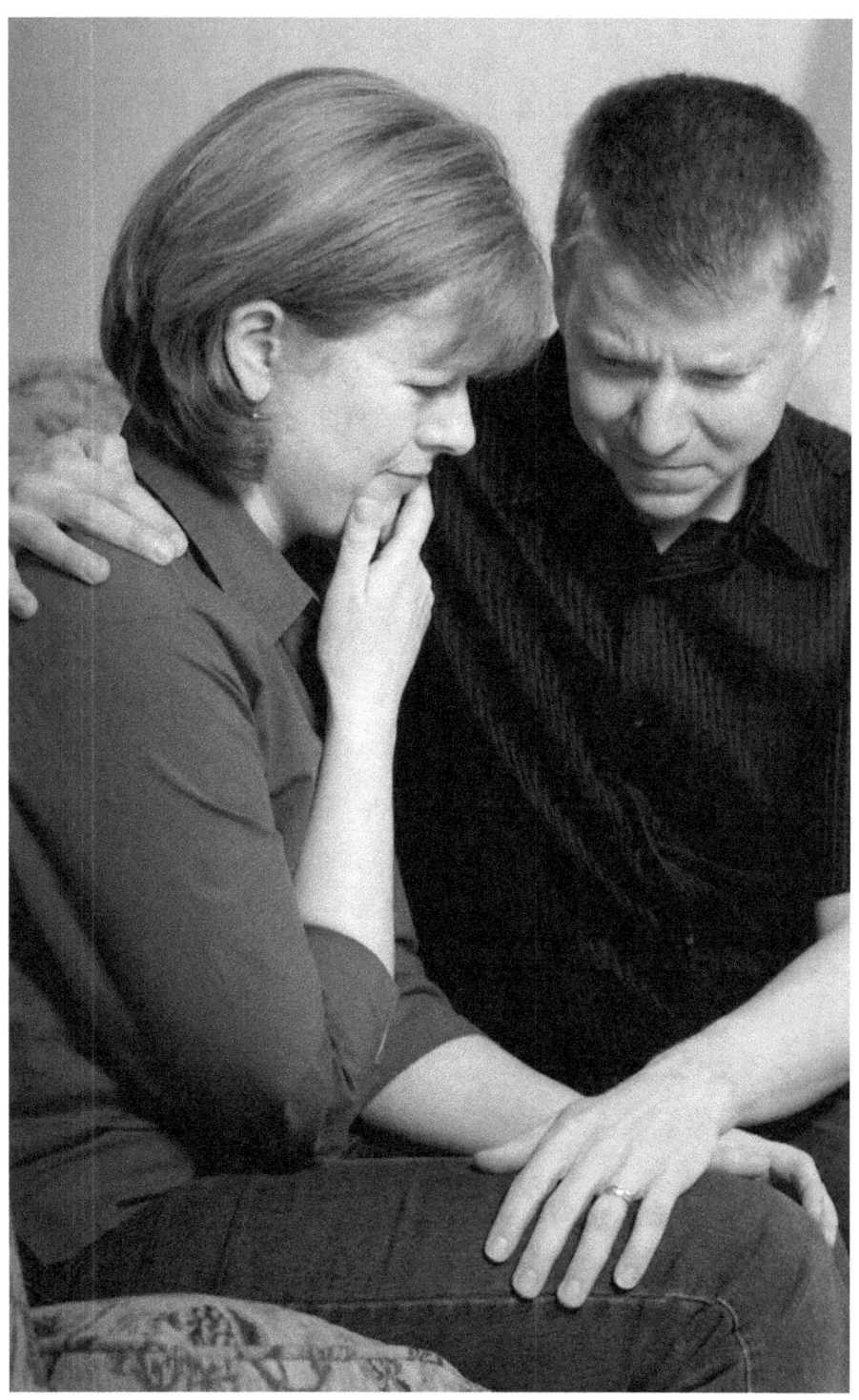

REFLUX VS. GASTROESOPHAGEAL REFLUX DISEASE (GERD)

GER occurs when pressure inside the stomach is higher than the pressure inside the esophagus. In normal GER, it is important that the pressure inside the stomach is higher than normal after external force is applied such as sitting or mobile activity or internal forces due to large-volume ingestion.

GERD is distinguished from GER by its association with damage to the esophageal lining and inflammation as consequence of the release of gastric content. The gastric content (gastric acid) has a low pH, and prolonged contact of any natural surface (in this case the mucosal lining of the esophagus) with the digestive enzymes that are present in gastric acid that leads to tissue damage and inflammation. It is well known that the oral cavity, teeth, airways (upper and lower respiratory tract systems), and esophagus can be affected by the caustic effects of digestive enzymes and gastric acid if the natural anti-reflux mechanisms do not perform optimally or fail to function entirely.

Our anti-reflux mechanisms consist of a small ring of muscle known as the lower esophageal sphincter, esophageal clearance (acid swiped back into the stomach), mucus, bicarbonate and saliva secretions from the mouth, and the esophageal lining. Additional mechanisms such as the upper esophageal sphincter, vocal cord reflex, and cough reflex help to protect the oral cavity and airways.

A combination of mechanisms work together to prevent the development of GERD: (a) gravity force, which is strongly exerted when a person is in an upright position, (b) muscle function from moving the food down the gastrointestinal stream in combination with the maintenance of high muscle tone at sphincter areas, and (c) the neutralizing function of bicarbonate, mucous, and saliva secretion which buffer or balance the acidic pH of gastric acid, preventing future damage. Other important mechanisms of reflux protection, primarily apnea and coughing, are located in the respiratory system and promote lung protection to avoid atypical GERD symptoms such as chronic cough, brochospasm, or pneumonia.

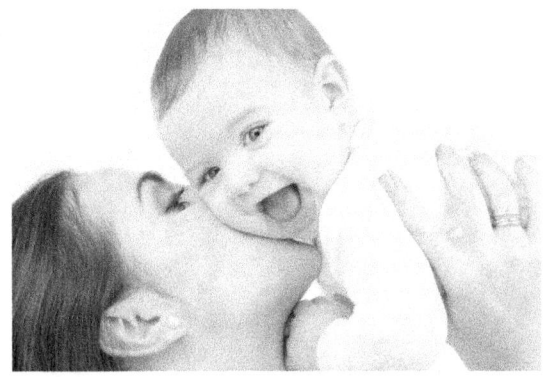

REFLUX FROM BIRTH TO WALKING

REFLUX IS SO COMMON in infancy that virtually all infants experience it to some degree. When these symptoms are very frequent and associated with medical symptoms, it is considered GERD. Over half of all infants experience GERD. This frequent reflux improves after the infant reaches one year of age, when the volume of food they need to grow decreases, they begin to eat more solids, and they master vertical positions like sitting or standing.

What are the risk factors for early childhood reflux?

Children are at increased risk for both GER and GERD, but all children, adolescents, or adults who suffer from one or more of anti-reflux preventive mechanisms not properly working will have a higher risk of GER. In general, neurologically-impaired children positioned horizontally or suffering from poor muscle tone or coordination, increasing intra-gastric pressure, will have a higher risk of reflux. Poor intestinal motility also will increase intra-gastric pressure and induce reflux, as will anatomical defects or surgical interventions such as esophageal atresias repair, trachea-esophageal fistulas repair, or the presence of a hiatal (diaphragm hiatus) hernia. Obesity and chronic lung disease are frequently observed in children with a higher degree of reflux.

DIAGNOSTIC TESTING FOR GERD

THE FIRST THING TO consider when diagnosing GERD is whether symptoms are present, what type(s) of symptoms are present, the intensity of the symptoms present, and the nutritional status of the individual. Careful analysis of symptoms may lead to a clear diagnosis from the outset.

POSSIBLE SYMPTOMS:

- Regurgitation, vomiting, or hematemesis (vomiting with blood)

- Poor weight gain

- Heartburn

- Chest pain

- Abdominal pain

- Irritability

- Protective positioning adopted by a child

- Anemia

- Asthma

- Wheezing

- Chronic cough

- Acute life-threatening events such as apnea

- Recurrent pneumonia

- Feeding refusal

- Sleep apnea

- Hoarseness

- Sinusitis

- Otitis media

- Dental erosions

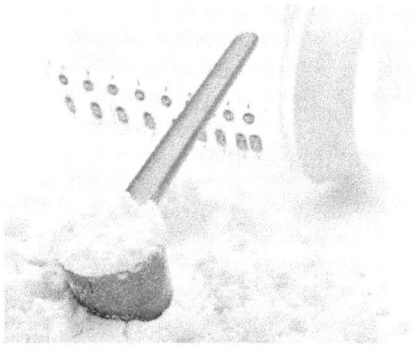

Evaluating the amount of food a child consumes and the speed of at which they are growing is critically important in diagnosing children. The volume eaten in relation to the child's weight should be appropriate to prevent GERD and induce appropriate weight gain (0.5 to 0.6 oz per kg q 3 hours). A higher volume of feeding will induce increased intra-gastric pressure and vomiting. The normal speed of growth for infants is a doubling of birth weight by six months with few exceptions, though a very limited number of infants double their birth weight at four months and are still considered normal. Infants at a normal growth rate then triple their weight by twelve months and quadruple their weight by twenty-four months. If growth occurs at a faster rate, the infant may be subject to overfeeding and an increased risk of GERD.

GASTROESOPHAGEAL REFLUX EVALUATION

Upper Gastrointestinal Studies: the main role of this radiological study is to evaluate potential defects in the gastrointestinal system which could lead to a predisposition to GERD, such as hiatal hernia, dilated esophagus, trachea-esophageal fistulas, sides of stomach and stomach position. This test may document instances of GER but will not provide conclusive evidence to diagnose GERD.

Esophageal pH Monitoring: this non-radiological study allows an evaluation of the level of acidity in the esophagus. This test will calculate the number of episodes in which the esophageal pH is less than four, and the duration of episodes of low pH over twenty-four hours, in order to calculate a reflux index. This test is very sensitive and can associate reflux with esophagitis or significant reflux. The downside of esophageal pH monitoring is that it cannot detect reflux episodes that are not acidic, and during the test anti-reflux medication needs to be withheld until the study is completed.

Esophageal Electrical Impedance Monitoring: this technology measures the current generated by the lining of the esophageal mucosa when they are close to each other. The impedance change along the length of the mucosal lining allows doctors to see the direction of bolus movement if the bolus is up (reflux) or down (swallowing). This enables the diagnosis of reflux and the size of reflux with no need to measure changes of pH; in others words it is not limited to acidic reflux. Impedance technology and pH monitoring are powerful tools to analyze acidic versus non-acidic reflux, the size of the reflux, and associated symptoms.

Upper Endoscopy with Biopsy: this technology allows the gastroenterologist to evaluate the degree of damage caused by reflux and to distinguish reflux disease from other diseases. It also allows the evaluation of additional risk factors for GERD, or complications from GERD such as Barrett's esophagus or strictures.

Laryngoscopy: this is a direct or indirect visualization of the pharynx, and it is limited to situations in which there are upper respiratory symptoms such as hoarseness, recurrent sinusitis, cough, and pneumonia. The interpretation of observations is operator dependent.

Bronchoscopy: this tool looks for evidence of gastric content located in the bronchus or lungs, and it is documented by the presence of lipid-laden macrophages

Scintigraphy or Gastric Emptying Scan with Twenty-four-hour-delayed Pictures: after ingesting a radio-labeled food, multiple pictures are taken every twenty minutes to detect the presence of food above the stomach. Delayed pictures are used to see if there is food in the lungs after sleeping overnight

Trial of Anti-reflux Therapy or Empiric Therapy: this approach can be used when clinical presentation is highly suggestive of GERD and a short therapy should be considered with close monitoring of the response of the symptoms to the anti-reflux medication.

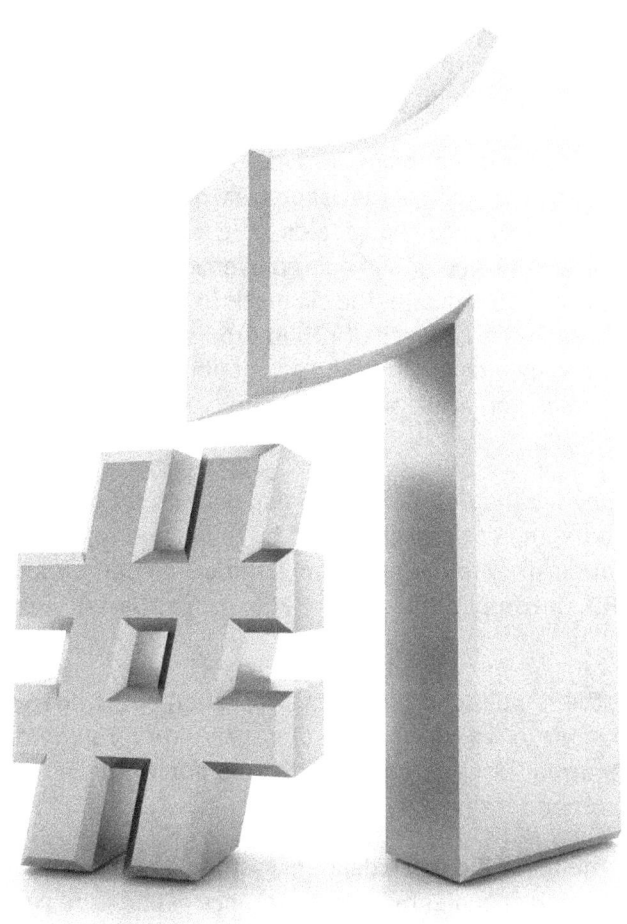

TREATMENT FOR RELUX

Reflux disease treatment depends upon the symptoms and degree of reflux. The reflux treatment is focused on decreasing symptoms, prevention of damage, and avoidance of the complications of GER.

The first goal of reflux therapy should be to focus on feeding volume and to schedule feeding-time intervention. Infants should drink from 0.5 to 0.6 oz/kg (0.25 to 0.27 oz/lb) per feeding, which should occur every 3 hours during the first 6 months then decrease to every 3.5 hours from the ages of 6 to 12 months. It is important to appreciate that feeding an infant every 3 hours provides a total of 8 feedings per day, which is a big difference from feeding every 2 hours which provides 12 feedings per day, leaving the infant ingesting 15 to 20 % more than recommended. It is also important to ensure that all caregivers understand and follow the scheduled recommendations.

NON-PHARMACOLOGIC TREATMENT

Non-pharmacologic options for GERD therapy in infants include:

Infant Bottles: There are many types and shapes of baby bottles. The best infant bottle is know as **Dr. Spinetti's Perfect Feeding**™©® infant bottle. This Bottle has a medical designed feeding scale, this scale converts one unique infant feature, the baby's weight, to the correct amount of formula deliver to the infant per feeding and estimate correct the infant stomach size.

This bottle is now available at Pediatric Gastroenterology clinic of South Texas

www.pgcost.com and Email: info@pgcost.com

Positioning Changes: up to a 45 degree angle for 45 to 60 minutes after eating. The American Academy of Pediatrics still recommends the supine position for sleeping, because this reduces the rate of sudden infant death when compared to other sleeping positions. A lateral position may also be used for sleeping, but the prone position should never be used.

Formula Changes: thickening an infant's formula with rice cereal is appropriate after birth to control GERD. A concentration range of 1 tbs of rice cereal per 2 oz of formula to 1 tbs of rice cereal per 1 oz of formula should be appropriate. This is done by carefully and minimally cutting the tip of a bottle nipple into a cross in order to allow for the thicker formula. The use of hypoallergenic formulas has been documented to help with formula allergy, which can induce GERD, and also helps reduce the time that the formula stays inside the stomach. Further reduction in the volume with an increase in concentration of calories in the child's formula (increase to 22 or 24 cal/oz) may also be appropriate. Increasing the volume of feeding should be done at a rate of no more than 0.25 oz every 1 to 2 weeks. The amount of breast-feeding provided an infant should take into consideration the level of maternal breast milk produced and kept to an average maximum of 10 to 15 minutes total every 3 hours.

Eating Habits: in children and adolescents large amounts of food and frequent feeding could induce GERD. In addition, large volumes of liquid should be avoided as well as sugar and artificial sweeteners, as they may induce pain and GERD. A good rule of thumb is for children aged 10 years and younger to limit themselves to 4.5 oz volume 5 times a day, and for children older than 10 years to 5 to 6 oz volume 5 times per day in addition to their regular diet.

Water breaks for sport participants should be limited to 3 to 4 oz of water every 20 to 30 minutes during the first hour of exercise and in subsequent hours the participants may alternate with sports drinks at the same volume and frequency.

*Special Note: it is important to avoid food items recognized to induce GERD such as fatty foods, chocolate, peppermint, and carbonated drinks. Maintenance of a healthy weight is important in prevention and treatment of reflux. Also treatment of constipation is a well-known additional intervention.

PHARMACOLOGIC TREATMENT

A number of pharmacologic treatment approaches for GER are known and include:

Acid Damage Prevention: oral antacids and sucralfate are well-known therapies for GER and are very effective in relieving its painful symptoms. These should be used on an as-needed basis due to their secondary effects which may occur with prolonged use. Antacids will buffer the excess gastric acid, and sucralfate will cover the mucosa to help in the process of healing.

Agents that Alter Gastrointestinal Motility: these agents, also known as prokinetic agents, are controversial in terms of efficacy and side effects. These agents work by increasing the mobility of food through the gastric system, which reduces the chances of reflux. Erythromycin is an antibiotic which has been well documented to improve motility and prevent reflux in specific circumstances.

Acid Suppression: these agents act by inhibiting the secretion of excess acid in the stomach, reducing the damaging effects of reflux. Examples of these drugs include H2-receptor antagonists (H2RAs), which act to decrease acid secretion by inhibiting the histamine-2 receptor on gastric parietal cells that are responsible aiding secretion in the stomach. H2RA agents include Cimetidine, Ranitidine, Nizatidine, and Famotidine. Proton pump inhibitors (PPIs) covalently bind and deactivate the H+, K+ ATPase pumps in the stomach, providing more effective gastric acid suppression compared to H2RAs. Omeprazole, Lansoprazole, Pantoprazole and Esomeprazole are examples of PPIs.

*The best way to administer a PPI is 30 minutes to 1 hour before breakfast in a single dose to maximize acid suppression after breakfast. Atypical GERD (respiratory symptoms), persistence of symptoms, or Barrett's esophagus will require a second PPI dose thirty minutes to 1 hour before dinner time. In children medication refusal could be avoided by using a dissolvable dose or opening the capsule and diluting it in 10 cc of fruit juice or apple sauce.

Acid-suppression medication is an excellent therapeutic approach for GERD, but using the medications for prolonged periods often leads to an increased risk of gastrointestinal and respiratory infections, vitamin B12 deficiency, and osteopenia with fractures.

SURGICAL TREATMENT

It is possible to perform anti-reflux surgery in select groups of patients. Anti-reflux therapy should first focus on managing the non-medical causes of GERD; if conditions persist, a medical option should be considered, leaving surgery as the final option because of its associated complications.

Nissen Fundoplication: is the most commonly performed surgical procedure for GERD in which the upper part of the stomach is wrapped, or plicate, around the lower end of the esophagus and stitched in place, reinforcing the closing function of the lower esophageal sphincter. The Nissen fundoplication is an excellent surgery when properly indicated; however, this is not a complication-free procedure and is much more difficult to reverse once a complication is presented.

Complications from the Nissen fundoplication arise from being too tight or too loose, nerve entrapment and its subsequent dysmotility which leads to slow gastric emptying, gas bloating syndrome which leads to accelerated gastric emptying (dumping syndrome), and anatomic modification of the gastric outlet while pulling the wrap which induces gastric outlet obstruction.

Future technologies such as endoscopic surgery have yet to be proven effective.

CYCLIC VOMITING SYNDROME AND ABDOMINAL MIGRAINE SYNDROME

CYCLIC VOMITING SYNDROME. THERE was a time I never imagined that this rare illness existed, but the past years have taught me how to treat my little daughter's crises.

There were times when her crises would begin with very strong headaches. One day it came so violently that her school called me to pick her up. She kept vomiting and was suffering from a very strong headache; she even had a fever. The school nurse was scared and wanted to call an ambulance, but I took her home, gave her a bath with warm water, administered a dose of medicine for her severe vomiting as well as a dose for her pain, and she fell into a deep sleep. I still keep her room as dark and cool as possible for these occasions. At around seven that evening, she woke up and told me she was hungry. I started her recovery by giving her broth and juice. The next day she looked better, but she still felt compelled to vomit, and she couldn't stop trembling. Her headache was not as intense; I kept her home; I bathed her and continued to hydrate her all day. On the third day, she started eating more. She was in a better mood, and she was able to go to school.

However, my daughter's crises aren't always the same. On one of the many occasions that we had to go to the hospital, her crisis took a somewhat different path. She woke up at five in the morning with a debilitating stomachache and headache. She was shaking, pale, and repeatedly vomiting. I still remember calling her doctor and immediately having her admitted to the hospital. She was placed in the intensive care unit, where my daughter was found to be dehydrated. She slept for a day and a half. On the morning of the second day, my daughter turned red. I called the nurse so she could check her temperature which turned out to be normal; the nurse voiced that it was strange that my daughter did not have a high temperature or fever given how flushed she was. The nurse changed the thermometer, but it measured the same temperature. After about one hour, my daughter turned pale and began saying, "Mommy, take the hot rocks off my back. They aren't letting me rest." Her words left me speechless. Her leg also hurt her a lot.

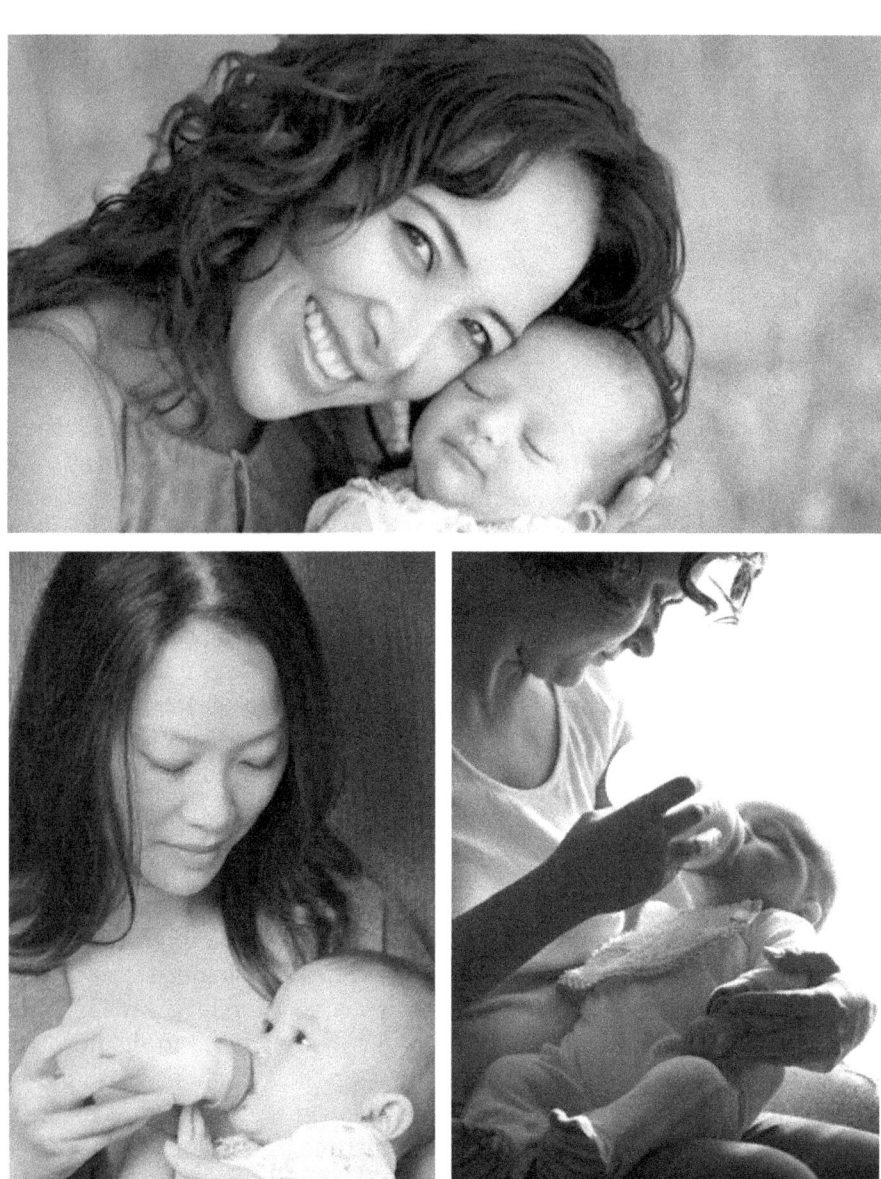

CYCLIC VOMITING SYNDROME

CYCLIC VOMITING SYNDROME IS a very characteristic phenomenon in which patients present with recurrent episodes of vomiting, which are usually severe and occasionally incapacitating, preventing the patient from performing his/her standard activities. An episode usually requires a medical evaluation, which then usually results in a negative work up. The vomiting usually stops quickly and is often followed by completely asymptomatic periods of time. During these periods, patients appear completely healthy and are able to perform their standard activities.

These patients are usually provided a series of wrong diagnoses, often including recurrent gastroenteritis, virus illness, and recurrent strep throat. Diagnoses may also include psychiatric disorders such as depression, bipolar disorder, and many others. The reoccurrence of the alternating pattern of illness and no illness can range from a few times a week to few times a year.

The symptomatic periods are very specific and usually called stereotyped:

In children the symptoms of cyclic vomiting syndrome present suddenly with a lack of appetite, change in behavior, irritability, sleepiness, change of skin color (often the child's face turns pale or paleness centers around the mouth), facial flushing, occasionally increased temperature or high fever, sweating, headache, abdominal pain (pain throughout the chest and abdominal cavity), and recurrent and frequent retching and vomiting of food initially, which rapidly changes to a yellow or green (bilious) color with occasional traces of blood (hematemesis). The first few stools are soft, loose or full of mucous, and occasionally the child's skin will tingle with a feeling of ants moving over their skin or areas suffering from hot or burning sensations. The symptomatic period follows its own course and may last from a few minutes up to seven days.

After following its course, symptoms are often suddenly resolved, and the child is able to perform his/her regular activities.

Cyclic vomiting syndrome is most frequently seen in children and adolescents from five to fifteen year of age, but early cases and older patients are also diagnosed at a lower frequency. Cyclic vomiting syndrome is a diagnosis of exclusion, and its specific etiology or reason has yet to be elucidated. But it is clearly associated with neuron-intestinal dysfunction with multiple triggers for the symptoms.

One of the most prominent current theories is that this dysfunction is triggered by serotonin which can cause a cascade of symptoms, from migraines to flushed skin, from smooth muscle contraction from small vascular vessels to intestinal wall or any other intra-abdominal viscera. These symptoms could result in poor blood flow to the bowel, leading to spasms that induce the severe pain, vomiting, and changes in behavior described above.

Due to the severity of the symptoms, other important diagnoses should be evaluated before cyclical vomiting disorder is determined.

These include:

- Intracranial tumors, sinusitis, and any cranial infection otitis media.

- Gastrointestinal peptic ulcer disease, duodenal ulcers, intestinal malrotation or distal obstruction, and pancreatitis including early appendicitis.

- Metabolic amino acid disorder, mitochondrial defect, and porphyria.

In our experience the most common diagnosis as secondary is after migraine, is sinusitis, duodenitis and infrequently follows inborn errors of metabolism.

Once the most important diagnoses are excluded and cyclic vomiting syndrome is considered, it is important to know that the most common trigger for episodes is stress of any kind, including extreme hot and cold temperatures, school tests, physical education or sports, large social gatherings, holidays, and familial problems. Specific foods, usually the same foods associated with migraines, may also trigger the symptoms. These food triggers include chocolate, soy, and dairy products.

This evaluation of these children can usually point to migraine, recurrent abdominal pain with nausea or frequent episodes of dizziness and nausea (less degree of headache).They have a strong family history of headache and migraines and irritable bowel syndrome as well as current family members.

After identifying symptoms and excluding other important diagnoses, therapy is focused on tracking and avoiding triggers such as stress and protecting patients from extreme weather changes.

Very useful pieces of advice in the handling of cyclic vomiting syndrome are:

- Follow a migraine diet or avoid foods that may trigger episodes.

- Avoid environmental triggers.

- Consider a regimen of cyproheptadine medication to prevent migraines in children (other migraine prevention medications are Propranolol, Topamax, and Aminotryptiline).

- Implement a regimen of acetaminophen at standard dose for body weight.

- Give the child warm, fifteen-minute baths.

- Consider applying warm compresses on the child's abdomen.

- Consult a doctor about antispasmodic medication.

- If vomiting becomes severe, Ondasentron (Zofran) may be very useful.

- Very often children suffering from cyclic vomiting syndrome become dehydrated because of a lack of appetite and vomiting. If this occurs, the child should be hospitalized immediately.

- Ensure the child receives enough sleep.

- Make sure the child is fed properly and frequently.

- A short trial of steroids as two to three single doses (in very severe cases)

ABDOMINAL MIGRAINES

———◆◆◆———

ABDOMINAL MIGRAINES ARE SIMILAR to cyclic vomiting syndrome but are accompanied by less severe symptoms that last a shorter duration. The major differences are that abdominal migraines do not cause severe and frequent vomiting, listless or sleepiness is less intense, and abdominal pain is less severe. However, the other symptoms of cyclic vomiting syndrome could be present during abdominal migraines.

A symptom-free period alternating with a symptomatic period as well as the stereotype group of symptoms (change of behavior, irritability, listlessness, changes in skin color, nausea, occasionally vomiting, headache, or dizziness) followed by symptom-free periods.

The prophylaxis and therapy is usually the same but secondary etiology such as sinusitis, peptic ulcer disease, should be excluded.

Cyproheptadine, Propranolol, and Topamax could be used as prophylactic therapy for abdominal migraine.

Tylenol, ibuprofen, or Excedrin could be used as abortive, stronger migraine medication as Sumatriptan should be use under medical supervision from neurologist.

Abortive migraine medication (Tylenol) and warm showers are very useful as well as local abdominal warm compresses.

VERY USEFUL PIECES OF ADVICE ARE:

Follow a migraine diet or avoid food and environmental triggers.

Cyproheptadine medication to prevent migraine in children.

Other migraine prevention medications are Propranolol, Topamax, and Aminotryptiline.

Acetaminophen at standard dose for body weight with a warm bath for fifteen minutes.

Consider warm compress in the abdomen.

Antispasmodic medication could be considered.

MIGRAINE PREVENTION DIET

Elimination of chocolate, caffeine, cheese, and other foods containing yogurt, sour cream, buttermilk, soy products, soy sauce, red wine vinegar and balsamic vinegar.

Avoidance of the following foods:

Apple and juice and cider.

Bananas.

Citrus fruits and juice.

Papaya and juice.

Passion fruit and juice.

Pears and juice.

Dried fruit, Grapes and juice.

Peas and Beans (fava, lima, navy, broad beans, lentils).

Tomato Onions Pickles Relish.

Canned and processed vegetables.

ALL cured, smoked, canned, pickled, or aged fish Anchovies Caviar Sardines.

ALL cured, smoked, canned, pickled, or aged meats.

Bacon (including beef, pork, and turkey).

Beef (all cured, smoked, canned, pickled, or aged).

Beef jerky.

Bologna of any kind.

Corned beef.

Deli meats (cured or smoked).

Ham (canned, cured, smoked, pickled, or aged).

Hot dogs (including chicken, turkey, and soy).

Liver and liverwurst.

Organ meats (such as kidneys or liver).

Pastrami.

Diet beverages/products that use the artificial sweetener aspartame (also known as NutraSweet and Soft drinks (Red Bull, Mountain Dew, Coke, and Equal).

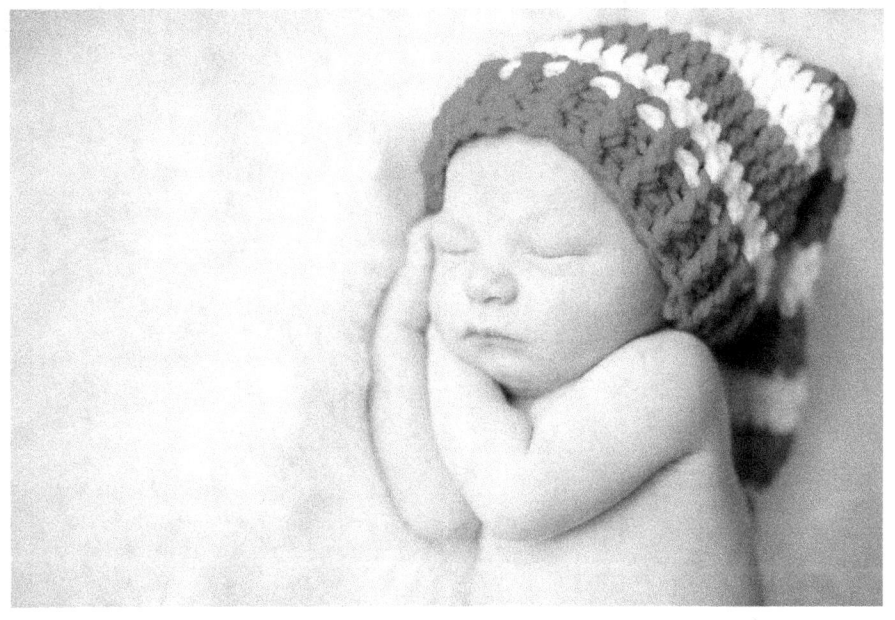

www.ingramcontent.com/pod-product-compliance
Lightning Source LLC
Chambersburg PA
CBHW070122010626
45794CB00012B/1237